Table of Contents

COPD is a killer – the third leading cause of death in the U.S. The National Institutes of Health states that, "COPD has no cure yet, and doctors don't know how to reverse the damage to the airways and lungs. However, treatments and lifestyle changes can help you feel better, stay more active, and slow the progress of the disease."

COPD is one of the most frustrating health issues that people deal with. It's very disabling, as reduced lung function makes it impossible to handle normal activities. To make matters worse, those afflicted with COPD may also have one or more other chronic illnesses. Most of those with COPD have emphysema and chronic bronchitis, both included under the general term COPD. Over time, the airways narrow, making it more difficult to breathe. Emphysema refers to damage to the walls between many of the air sacs in the lungs. Instead of many tiny air sacs, the person now has fewer, larger air sacs. This reduces gas exchange within the lungs. In other words, the lung's ability to take in oxygen and remove carbon dioxide is far less than is needed for proper breathing and good health. There is not enough oxygen and too much carbon dioxide.

Chronic bronchitis refers to the lining of the airways being always irritated and inflamed. The lining gets thicker; thick mucus makes it hard to breath.

Planning what you eat and balancing your meals are important ways to manage your health. Eating healthfully often means making changes in your current eating habits. Changing your eating habits will not cure COPD, but it can help you feel better. A registered dietitian can provide in-depth nutrition guidance, tailor educational information to meet your needs, and help you create and follow a personal action plan.

If you have COPD, why is good nutrition so important

Food is the fuel your body needs to perform all activities, including breathing. Your body uses food for energy as part of a process called metabolism. During metabolism, food and oxygen are changed into energy and carbon dioxide. You use energy for all of your activities - from sleeping to exercising.

Food provides your body with nutrients (carbohydrates, fat, and protein) that affect how much energy you will have and how much carbon dioxide is produced. Carbon dioxide is a waste product that leaves your body when you breathe out (exhale). If there is too much carbon dioxide in your body, you might feel weak. Breathing requires more energy for people with chronic obstructive pulmonary disease (COPD). The muscles used in breathing might require 10 times more calories than those of a person without COPD. Good nutrition helps the body fight infections. Chest infections are illnesses that often lead to hospitalization for people with COPD, so it is important to reduce your risk of infection by following a healthy diet.

Maintain a healthy body weight. Ask your healthcare provider or registered dietitian what your "goal" weight should be and how many calories you should consume per day.

If you are overweight, your heart and lungs have to work harder, making breathing more difficult. In addition, the extra weight might demand more oxygen. To achieve your ideal body weight, exercise regularly and limit your total daily calories. In contrast, being underweight might make you feel weak and tired, and might make you more likely to get an infection. People with COPD use more energy while breathing than the average person. Therefore, the pulmonary (breathing) muscles in someone with COPD might require up to 10 times the calories needed by a person without COPD. It is important for you to consume enough calories to produce energy in order to prevent wasting or weakening of the diaphragm and other pulmonary muscles.

Monitor your weight. Weigh yourself once or twice a week, unless your doctor recommends weighing yourself more often. If you are taking diuretics (water pills) or steroids, such as prednisone, you should weigh yourself daily since your weight might change. If you have an unexplained weight gain or loss (2 pounds in one day or 5 pounds in one week), contact your doctor. He or she might want to change your food or fluid intake to better manage your condition.

Drink plenty of fluids. You should drink at least 6 to 8 glasses (eight ounces each glass) of non-caffeinated beverages each day to keep mucus thin and easier to cough up. Limit caffeine (contained in coffee; tea; several carbonated beverages such as cola and Mountain Dew; and chocolate) as it might interfere with some of your medicines.

Some people with COPD who also have heart problems might need to limit their fluids, so be sure to follow your doctor's guidelines.

Include high-fiber foods — such as vegetables, fruits, cooked dried peas and beans (legumes), whole-grain cereals, pasta, and rice. Fiber is the indigestible part of plant food. Fiber helps move food along the digestive tract, better controls blood glucose levels, and might reduce the level of cholesterol in the blood.

The goal for everyone is to consume 20 to 35 grams of fiber each day. An example of what to eat in one day to help you get enough fiber includes: eating 1 cup of all-bran cereal for breakfast, a sandwich with two slices of whole-grain bread and 1 medium apple for lunch, and 1 cup of peas, dried beans, or lentils at dinner.

Control the sodium (salt) in your diet. Eating too much salt causes the body to keep or retain too much water, causing breathing to be more difficult. In addition to removing the salt shaker from your table:

• Use herbs or no-salt spices to flavor your food.

• Don't add salt to foods when cooking.

• Read food labels and avoid foods with more than 300 mg sodium/serving.

• Before using a salt substitute check with your doctor. Salt substitutes might contain other ingredients that can be just as harmful as salt.

• Make sure you are getting enough calcium and Vitamin D to keep your bones healthy. Good sources of these nutrients are foods made from milk (milk, cheese, yogurt, ice cream, and pudding) and foods fortified with calcium and Vitamin D. You may need to take calcium and Vitamin D supplements. Maintaining a healthy weight and exercising will also help with keeping bones healthy.

• Wear your cannula while eating if continuous oxygen is prescribed. Since eating and digestion require energy, your body will need the oxygen.

Avoid overeating and foods that cause gas or bloating. A full stomach or bloated abdomen might make breathing uncomfortable. Avoid the foods that cause gas or bloating. Some foods that cause gas for some people include:

• Carbonated beverages

• Fried, greasy, or heavily spiced foods

• Apples, avocados, and melons

• Beans, broccoli, Brussels sprouts, cabbage, cauliflower, corn, cucumbers, leeks, lentils, onions, peas, peppers, pimentos, radishes, scallions, shallots, and soybeans

Follow your doctor's other dietary guidelines. If you take diuretics (water pills), you might also need to increase your potassium intake. Some foods high in potassium include oranges, bananas, potatoes, asparagus, and tomatoes.

If you are short of breath while eating or right after meals, try these tips

• Clear your airways at least one hour before eating.

• Eat more slowly. Take small bites and chew your food slowly, breathing deeply while chewing. Try putting your utensils down between bites.

• Choose foods that are easy to chew.

• Try eating five or six small meals a day instead of three large meals. This will keep your stomach from filling up too much so your lungs have more room to expand.

• Try drinking liquids at the end of your meal. Drinking before or during the meal might make you feel full or bloated.

• Eat while sitting up to ease the pressure on your lungs.

• Use pursed-lip breathing.

• Eat a variety of foods from all the food groups to get the nutrients you need. The recommended number of servings per day are listed below. These guidelines are for a 2,000-calorie diet.

Grains

• Eat whole-grain cereals, breads, crackers, rice, or pasta every day.

• 1 oz. is about 1 slice of bread, 1 cup of cereal, or a half cup of cooked rice, cereal, or pasta.

• Eat 6 oz daily.

Vegetables

• Eat more dark green veggies like broccoli and more orange veggies like carrots.

• Eat more dry beans and peas like pinto beans and lentils.

• Eat 2.5 cups daily.

Fruits

• Eat a variety of fresh fruit.

• Choose fresh, frozen, canned or dried fruit.

• Go easy on fruit juices.

• Eat 2 cups daily.

Milk

• Choose low-fat or fat-free milk, yogurt, and other milk products.

• If you don't or can't consume milk, choose lactose-free products or calcium-fortified foods or beverages.

• Have 3 cups daily.

Meat and Beans

• Choose low-fat or lean meats and poultry. Bake it broil it, or grill it.

• Vary your protein routine-choose more fish, beans, peas, nuts, and seeds.

• Eat 5.5 oz. daily.

• If you are often too tired to eat later in the day, here are some guidelines:

• Choose foods that are easy to prepare. Save your energy for eating, otherwise you might be too tired to eat.

• Ask your family to help with meal preparations.

• Check to see if you are eligible to participate in your local Meals on Wheels program.

• Freeze extra portions of what you cook so you have a quick meal when you're too tired.

• Rest before eating so you can enjoy your meal.

• Try eating your main meal early in the day so you have enough energy to last you for the day.

Tips for improving your appetite

General guidelines

• Talk to your doctor. Sometimes, poor appetite is due to depression, which can be treated. Your appetite is likely to improve after depression is treated.

• Avoid non-nutritious beverages such as black coffee and tea.

• Try to eat more protein and fat, and less simple sugars.

• Eat small, frequent meals and snacks.

• Walk or participate in light activity to stimulate your appetite.

• Keep food visible and within easy reach.

Meal guidelines

• Drink beverages after a meal instead of before or during a meal so that you do not feel as full.

• Plan meals to include your favorite foods.

• Try eating the high-calorie foods in your meal first.

• Use your imagination to increase the variety of food you're eating.

Snack guidelines

• Don't waste your energy eating foods that provide little or no nutritional value (such as potato chips, candy bars, colas, and other snack foods).

• Choose high-protein and high-calorie snacks.

• Keep non-perishable snacks visible and within easy reach.

Dining guidelines

• Make food preparation an easy task. Choose foods that are easy to prepare and eat.

• Make eating a pleasurable experience, not a chore.

• Liven up your meals by using colorful place settings.

• Play background music during meals.

• Eat with others. Invite a guest to share your meal or go out to dinner.

• Use colorful garnishes such as parsley and red or yellow peppers, to make food look more appealing and appetizing.

• Ask your doctor for specific guidelines regarding alcohol. Your doctor might tell you to avoid or limit alcoholic beverages. Alcoholic beverages do not have much nutritional value and can interact with the medicines you are taking, especially oral steroids. Too much alcohol might slow your breathing and make it difficult for you to cough up mucus.

Tips for gaining weight

Drink milk or try one of the "High Calorie Recipes" listed below instead of drinking low-calorie beverages.

Ask your doctor or dietitian about nutritional supple ments. Sometimes, supplements in the form of snacks, drinks (such as Ensure or Boost) or vitamins might be prescribed to eat between meals. These supplements help you increase your calories and get the right amount of nutrients every day. The combination of exercise and these supplements can help you gain weight.

• Avoid low-fat or low-calorie products unless you have been given other dietary guidelines. Use whole milk, whole milk cheese, and yogurt.

• Use the "Calorie Boosters" listed in this book to add calories to your favorite foods.

• Adding fresh or frozen fruit to your shakes can give you different consistencies and more variety.

• High-calorie snacks

• Ice cream

• Cookies

• Pudding

• Cheese

• Granola bars

• Custard

• Sandwiches

• Nachos with cheese

• Eggs

• Crackers with peanut butter

• Bagels with peanut butter or cream cheese

• Cereal with half and half

• Fruit or vegetables with dips

• Yogurt with granola

• Popcorn with margarine and parmesan cheese

• Bread sticks with cheese sauce

Calorie Boosters

If you are having difficulty maintaining a healthy weight, try some of these calorie boosters:

Food Item: Egg yolk or whole egg

• Suggested Use: Before cooking, add egg yolk or whole egg to foods such as meat loaf, rice pudding, or macaroni and cheese. (To prevent illness, avoid the use of uncooked eggs.)

• Food Item: Non-fat powdered milk or undiluted evaporated milk

• Suggested Use: Add to beverages (including milk) or to these foods: creamed soups, yogurt, scrambled eggs, casseroles, pudding, mashed potatoes, custard, gravies, hot cereal, and/or sauces.

• Food Item: Cream cheese or shredded, melted, sliced, cubed, or grated cheese

• Suggested Use: Add to sandwiches, snacks, casseroles, crackers, eggs, soups, toast, pasta, potatoes, rice or vegetables, or serve as a snack.

• Food Item: Vegetable oils, mayonnaise, butter, margarine, or sour cream

• Suggested Use: Add margarine or mayonnaise to sandwiches; add any of these items to bread, casseroles, soups, eggs, cooked cereals, pasta, potatoes, rice, vegetables, pudding.

• Food Item: Peanut butter (creamy or crunchy)

• Suggested Use: Spread on bread, crackers, apples, bananas, or celery. Or add to cereal, custard, cookies, or milk shakes.

• Food Item: Nut dust (grind any type of nuts in a blender or food processor)

• Suggested Use: Add to puddings, gravy, mashed potatoes, casseroles, salads, yogurt, cereals.

• Food item: Miscellaneous foods (limit to one serving per day)

Suggested Use:

• Add: sugar, jelly, jam preserves, honey, corn syrup, maple syrup

• To: hot cereal, cold cereal, fruit, fruit salad, sweet potatoes, winter squash

How does diet affect COPD

A well-balanced diet may help reduce inflammation in a person with COPD.

A healthful diet can help prevent or manage some of the adverse health effects of COPD, a lung condition characterized by airflow limitation that makes it hard to breathe. According to reviews in 2015, a healthful, well-balanced diet can have the following beneficial health effects in people with COPD:

• Reducing inflammation

• Maintaining and improving muscle strength

• Improving lung function

• Lowering metabolic and heart disease risk

Foods to eat

The American Lung Association recommend the following types of food for people who have COPD:

Complex carbohydrates

Complex carbohydrates contain long chains of sugar molecules. The body takes time to break down these molecules. As such, complex carbohydrates provide a relatively sustained release of energy.

Foods that contain complex carbohydrates include:

• Fresh fruit and starchy vegetables

• Whole grains

• Whole grain bread and pasta

• Beans and lentils

If a person with COPD wants to gain weight, eating a variety of complex carbohydrates alongside healthful sources of fat and protein can help.

Alternatively, if a person with COPD has extra body fat to lose, replacing refined carbohydrate sources with complex carbs, protein, and healthful fat can promote weight loss.

Fiber-rich foods

According to the American Lung Association, a person with COPD should aim for around 20–30 grams of fiber each day. Foods that contain a good amount of fiber include:

• Beans and lentils

• Fruits and vegetables

• Nuts and seeds

• Whole grains, such as oats

• Vegetables

• Protein

A study in the International Journal of Chronic Obstructive Pulmonary Disease found that people in Vietnam with COPD had increased protein needs. Including protein-rich foods at meals and snacks may help with improving nutritional status and quality of life.

Foods that are high in protein include

• Meat and poultry

• Fish

• Eggs

• Nuts and seeds

• Legumes

• Tofu

• Cheese

• Milk

Protein sources can help increase muscle mass and help people gain weight if needed. Alternatively, adding high-quality protein sources to meals and snacks or swapping refined carbohydrate sources with healthful proteins may promote weight loss.

Mono and polyunsaturated fats

Mono and polyunsaturated fats are healthful fats that can help lower a person's cholesterol. Some foods that contain these fats include:

• Certain vegetable oils, such as olive oil and avocado oil

• Certain fish, including salmon

• Nuts and seeds

• Avocados

According to the American Lung Association, a person with COPD who is looking to gain weight should try adding these fats to meals. If they are looking to lose weight, they should limit their intake of all fats, including mono and polyunsaturated fats.

Foods to avoid

The American Lung Association recommend that people with COPD avoid or limit the following food types:

Simple carbohydrates

Simple carbohydrates provide fewer nutrients than complex carbohydrates. Foods consisting of simple carbohydrates include:

• Table sugar

• Chocolate and candy

• Cakes and other sugary desserts

• Sugary drinks

• Processed foods

• White bread and pasta

Unhealthful fats

Many high-fat foods are nutritious, and people can include them in
a healthful diet. However, many highly processed foods are high-
fat, and people with COPD should avoid or limit them to promote
overall health.

People with COPD must avoid or limit the following high-fat foods:

• Fast food

• Bacon and other processed meats

• Fried foods

• Sugary pastries

• Margarine

• Ice cream

Some people with COPD may experience a lack of appetite due to breathing difficulties and general chest discomfort. Breathing difficulties also increase the physical effort required for eating, and this can make it difficult for a person to finish meals.

Below are some tips that may help improve a person's appetite and energy levels, or ease the effort required for eating.

Eating smaller meals: Instead of eating three large meals a day, it may be helpful to aim to eat four to six smaller meals. This should reduce stomach fullness and associated pressure on the lungs.

Eating the main meal earlier: A person may find that they have more energy throughout the day if they eat their main meal earlier in the day.

Drinks: A 2019 review found that readily available high-protein, high-energy drinks can help boost nutrition in people unable to tolerate high volumes of food.

COPD can lead to changes in a person's metabolism and body composition.

Changes in metabolism

Metabolism is the process that occurs within the body to sustain life, such as converting the food a person eats into energy.

A person who has COPD and hyper-metabolism will require more calories than someone who does not have these conditions.

Changes in body composition

Around 25-40% of people with COPD develop pulmonary cachexia syndrome (PCS). This is a metabolic condition that causes weight loss and muscle wasting.

Some factors that may contribute to PCS in COPD include:

• Widespread, or systemic, inflammation

• Hyper-metabolism and insufficient calorie intake

• Increased energy expenditure due to more effortful breathing

• Muscle atrophy resulting from inactivity

• Use of glucocorticoid medications to treat COPD

People with COPD and PCS typically require dietary interventions to counteract the PCS and prevent further health complications.

COPD and weight

People with COPD who have underweight or overweight may encounter additional health issues.

Being underweight can sometimes indicate malnutrition. A 2019 review notes that malnutrition alongside COPD may lead to poor health outcomes, including increased risk of COPD exacerbations or flare-ups. According to a 2013 review, people who have COPD with obesity tend to experience more significant breathing difficulties compared to people with COPD without obesity. According to the review, excess fat, or adipose tissue, puts pressure on the chest wall, exacerbating breathing difficulties.

A 2014 review suggests that controlling obesity may help prevent and manage lung impairment in people with COPD.

If a person with COPD is looking to gain or lose weight, they should discuss the necessary dietary and exercise requirements with their healthcare team.

COPD and exercise

According to a 2016 review, exercise can improve muscle function and exercise tolerance in people with COPD.

Another 2016 study found that exercise and dietary restriction provided additional benefits for participants who had COPD and obesity. These benefits included:

• Improved weight

• Improved exercise tolerance

• Improved health status

People with COPD who have underweight or have PCS may also benefit from regular exercise. If someone with COPD wishes to take up exercise, they should discuss this with their healthcare team.

Earth Clinic readers have told us that their favorite home remedy for COPD (Chronic Obstructive Pulmonary Disease) is the Hydrogen Peroxide Inhalation Method. Some readers experienced wonderful results with this natural remedy in as little as two weeks. In fact, for the past 10 years, Bill Munro's Hydrogen Peroxide Inhalation Method has been one of Earth Clinic's most popular natural cures for many different ailments. Other nebulizer treatments are helpful as well, such as DMSO, Colloidal Silver, and MSM.

Symptoms of COPD

You may have COPD and not know it. Over 24 million people in the U.S. have COPD, but more than HALF of those people do not know that they have this very serious problem. If you are experiencing these symptoms, get diagnosed and then take action before more damage is done to your lungs. Otherwise, COPD will continue to get worse, until you need to be attached to an oxygen tank in order to breathe at all.

Are you experiencing these symptoms?

Frequent coughing, with or without mucus;

Feeling out of breath more and more often;

Wheezing;

A tight feeling in the chest.

If you have COPD, more oxygen is just exactly what you need. Many Earth Clinic readers with COPD reported success following this method. The link above will show you exactly how to use Bill's method. Please do follow the instructions. Do not overdo on the "more is better" theory. It isn't. Both Bill and his wife safely inhaled hydrogen peroxide daily for at least 9 years, enjoying improved overall health. Their blood oxygen levels remained in the high 90s.

Normal blood oxygen levels are 95-100%.

Below 90% is considered hypoxemia, leading to an asthma crisis, sleep apnea, pulmonary infection, etc.

A blood oxygen level below 80% is a critical situation that could result in a damaged brain or heart; respiratory or cardiac arrest can occur at this level of low blood oxygen.

COPD and Viral and Bacterial Infections

The most common cause of COPD exacerbations is viruses, particularly the flu, rhinovirus or adenovirus. Mycoplasma and chlamydia are bacteria that can also be responsible for lung infections. These organisms cannot thrive in an oxygen-rich environment, such as that created by inhaling hydrogen peroxide following the suggested method.

If You Smoke, Quit!

Smoking is the leading cause of COPD. While there are other risk factors, such as pollution, second-hand smoke, family history or chemical fumes, smoking is the most important risk factor by a wide margin. Don't be one of the people sneaking into the garage for a cigarette and then hobbling back to the oxygen tank in order to get a breath of air. If you don't quit now, you will be forced to when you're totally bed-bound and cannot breathe at all without the oxygen tank. Our readers have sent in a lot of remedies that have helped them to quit smoking. We hope that one of their recommendations will help you.

Breathing comes to us naturally and (usually) pretty easily. However, if you have chronic obstructive pulmonary disease, better known as COPD, you have trouble doing what connects us to life – you can't easily breathe.

The disease can affect your airways, air sacs or both. It's the third leading cause of death in the United States, according to the American Lung Association – affecting more than 11 million Americans and another estimated 24 million who go undiagnosed.

If you were recently diagnosed with COPD, your mind may be spinning with questions like, "Can COPD be reversed?" or "Is COPD fatal or curable?" Pulmonologist Kathrin Nicolacakis, MD, sheds light on four common myths about COPD and why it's often misunderstood:

Myth 1: Only smokers get COPD

Fact: While COPD is often associated with smoking, and rightly so, there are a substantial number of people with this condition who never smoked.

According to the National Institutes of Health, 42% of COPD sufferers are former smokers, 34% are current smokers and the rest – which make up 24% — never lit a cigarette.

Myth 2: There's no treatment for COPD

Fact: There is a lot that can be done for COPD patients.

"People need to know that COPD is treatable, and if you have symptoms, there are many options to help you feel better," says Dr. Nicolacakis. "We may not be able to reverse it, but we can control the symptoms and prevent further damage to the lungs."

It's important to quit smoking, eat a healthy diet, get plenty of exercise and keep up on your influenza and pneumonia vaccines to prevent serious illness. Taking care of yourself in these ways, plus taking your medications, can sometimes help offset the complications of COPD.

Your doctor will help tailor medications to your needs. Medications include inhalers that open your airways or reduce airway inflammation, supplemental oxygen, and alpha-1-antitrypsin (A1AT) infusions if you have an inherited deficiency. PDE4 enzyme inhibitors can reduce inflammation in some patients, too.

Myth 3: If you have COPD, it's too late to quit smoking

Fact: "Some people think that once they are diagnosed with COPD, there's no benefit to quitting smoking," says Dr. Nicolacakis. "But it's never too late to quit because it will slow the progression of the disease."

You may wonder: Will COPD go away if I stop smoking?

Unfortunately, the lung damage that characterizes COPD is cumulative, which means that it doesn't go away just because you kicked the habit, but there's still a lot of benefit to quitting.

However, if you quit smoking early enough, near-normal lung function may return.

"Try a smoking cessation program," she says. "Combining nicotine replacement with counseling, group support and medication is your best chance of success."

Myth 4: Exercise is too hard if you have COPD

Fact: If you find that shortness of breath makes it too difficult to be physically active, there are further steps you can take. Talk to your doctor if they recommend pulmonary rehabilitation, where specialized respiratory therapists teach breathing techniques, exercises and proper nutrition to make living with COPD easier.

"Moderate exercise will not hurt your lungs, either," she says. "In fact, it can lessen COPD symptoms, strengthen your heart and reduce stress."

To get your body moving, build up to 20 to 30 minutes of exercise three to four times a week. Combine a safe cardiovascular activity you enjoy with stretching and strengthening exercises. While you're getting your workout in, be sure to breathe out slowly through pursed lips, taking twice as long to exhale as to inhale. Rest before and after exercise, and wait an hour and a half after meals to work out.

Tips to manage your COPD

If you have COPD, there are steps you can take so that living with it more manageable. Managing it well will allow you to stay active and involved with family and friends. Besides quitting smoking, taking prescribed medications and exercising, the following can also help:

Conserve your energy. Try to get plenty of sleep at night and plan for one rest period per day. Elevate your head at night and your feet during the day when your ankles swell. Also, rest before and after activities and make realistic plans for chores and avoid extreme exertion, such as heavy lifting, raking and shoveling. It's best to avoid working long days.

Prevent respiratory infections. Wash your hands carefully, especially after being outside. Get a flu shot six weeks before the start of flu season each year and get the pneumococcal vaccine every five years to help prevent pneumonia. See your doctor if you think you're getting sick and if they recommend antibiotics that can prevent serious chest infections.

Eat right. Maintain a healthy weight. If you're too heavy, your heart and lungs have to work too hard. If you're too thin, you're more easily fatigued and at higher risk of chest infections. Dr. Nicolacakis recommends drinking six to eight glasses of caffeine-free liquid every day to thin mucus in the airways and eating fiber to keep your digestion moving. It's important to limit salt to avoid water retention and bloating and to avoid overeating. If you get full too fast, consider five to six small meals a day, take small bites, and save liquids for the end of the meal. If you have an oxygen cannula, wear it while eating.

Recipes

High-calorie recipes to promote weight gain

If you are having difficulty maintaining a healthy weight, try some of these "Calorie Boosters."

Super Shake

Ingredients:

• 1 cup whole milk

• 1 cup ice cream (1-2 scoops)

• 1 package Carnation Instant Breakfast

Directions - Pour all ingredients into a blender. Mix well. Makes one serving; 550 calories per serving.

Chocolate Peanut Butter Shake

Ingredients:

• 1/2 cup heavy whipping cream

• 3 tablespoons creamy peanut butter

• 3 tablespoons chocolate syrup

• 1-1/2 cups chocolate ice cream

Directions - Pour all ingredients into a blender. Mix well. Makes one serving; 1090 calories per serving.

Super Pudding

Ingredients:

• 2 cups whole milk

• 2 tablespoons vegetable oil

• 1 package instant pudding

• 3/4 cup non-fat, dry milk powder

Directions - Blend milk and oil. Add pudding mix and mix well. Pour into dishes (1/2 cup servings). Makes four 1/2 cup servings; 250 calories per serving.

Great Grape Slush

Ingredients:

• 2 grape juice bars

• 1/2 cup grape juice or 7-up

• 2 tablespoons corn syrup

• 1 tablespoon corn oil

Directions - Pour all ingredients into a blender. Mix well. Makes one serving; 490 calories per serving.

Cucumber, Tomato and Onion Salad

Yield: 2 servings (7 servings of vegetables)

Ingredients

• 2 cucumbers, chunked

• 3 tomatoes, sliced

• 1 red onion, diced

• 2 ounces olive oil

• 1 ounce vinegar

• 1 teaspoon basil

• 1 teaspoon savory

• Salt and pepper to taste

Directions

• Toss all ingredients together. Let flavors mingle for an hour in the refrigerator. Serve cold.

• Onions are excellent for clearing out the lungs. Tomatoes are great for your vision, and cucumbers are beauty foods for your skin.

Rice Vegetable Salad

Yield: 3 servings (12 servings fruits/vegetables)

Ingredients

• 2 cups rice pilaf, cooked

• 1 ounce olive oil

• 2 cups shredded carrots

• 1 cup frozen peas

• ½ cup chopped celery

• 1 zucchini, chopped

• 1 cucumber, chopped

• 2 ounces sliced almonds

• 1 cup diced or chunked pineapple

• Salt and pepper

Directions

• Toss all ingredients together and add salt and pepper to taste.

• Pineapple is an excellent source of enzymes and bromelain, which is a painkiller. Celery is helpful as a diuretic and good for the heart. Almonds can help lower cholesterol.

Carrot Raisin Salad

Yield: 3 servings (9 servings fruits and vegetables)

Ingredients

• 3 cups shredded carrots

• ½ cup raisins

- 1 cup chopped celery

- ½ cup chopped parsley

- ½ cup chopped cilantro

- 2 tablespoons olive oil or coconut oil

- 1 tablespoon shredded coconut

- Juice of one lime

- ½ cup walnuts, chopped

Directions

- Toss all ingredients together and enjoy.

- Carrots are high in beta-carotene, which is beneficial for the lungs. Celery is a diuretic and helpful for the heart. Parsley is good for the kidney. Coconut has anti-microbial properties. Lime contains medicinal constituents that are anti-cancer.

• You could even make up these salads on Sunday for the week and then have them available for the rest of the week. It would make your meal preparation go a lot faster!

Apple Cider Vinegar for COPD

For people with chronic obstructive pulmonary disease (COPD), any natural remedy that can help manage COPD symptoms is highly sought after. This is where apple cider vinegar comes in. Apple cider vinegar contains many natural compounds that have antioxidant properties. The most potent of these compounds is acetic acid. The reason why these antioxidants are so beneficial is because they protect cells from free radicals that cause damage to cell DNA. These compounds in apple cider vinegar convert superoxide and other harmful free radicals into less harmful oxygen and hydrogen peroxide. Additionally, apple cider vinegar thins and virtually eliminates mucus build which is common with people who suffer from COPD.

The Apple Cider Vinegar for COPD Recipe

• 2 teaspoons apple cider vinegar

• 1/2 fresh lemon

• 8 oz warm water

Squeezed the juice from 1/2 lemon and combine with the apple cider vinegar and warm water. Drink this twice per day and enjoy the difference in how you feel!

Apple Cider Vinegar for Asthma

It might seem silly to you that ingesting vinegar would have anything to do with your ability to breathe, but apple cider vinegar is also a common remedy for acid reflux, a symptom of GERD, which is closely related to asthma in many cases. Airways in your esophagus may trigger to close because of acid and other symptoms of GERD including asthma-like hoarseness and chronic cough.

It is estimated that more than 75% of patients with asthma also experience gastroesophageal reflux disease (GERD). People with asthma are twice as likely to have GERD as those people who do not have asthma. Of those people with asthma, those who have a severe, chronic form that is resistant to treatment are most likely to also have GERD. The acidity in apple cider vinegar helps hydrochloric acid, or stomach acid, do its job which may be why apple cider vinegar relieves acid reflux, and therefore relieves asthma.

Ingredients

• 1 tablespoon apple cider vinegar

• 1 teaspoon of honey

• 1/2 cup warm water

Combine apple cider vinegar and honey in warm water. Sip this mixture when in you feel an asthma attack coming on.

Apple Cider Vinegar for Bronchitis

Apple cider vinegar contains acetic acid and probiotics that help cure bronchitis by balancing the pH levels in the body, therefore reducing inflammation and swelling. Adding honey to your apple cider vinegar drink is also beneficial. Honey is a natural demulcent that soothes the cough that occurs with bronchitis. Additionally, the antiviral, antibacterial, and anti-inflammatory properties of honey help reduce the swelling of the bronchial tubes. An apple cider vinegar and honey concoction work as an incredible expectorant to reduce the thickness of the mucus and expel the phlegm, thus relieving bronchitis.

Ingredients

• 1/4 cup Apple cider vinegar

• 1 tablespoon honey

• 2 cups of water

Combine the apple cider vinegar, honey, and water in a pitcher and stir until all ingredients are dissolved. Drink daily until your bronchitis symptoms are relieved.